Overcoming Depression for
By Tilly McIntyre – A Young Adult V
T-Sl

Copyright © 2014 by Tilly McIntyre

All rights reserved. No part of this publication may be reproduced, distributed, or transmitted in any form or by any means, including photocopying, recording, or other electronic or mechanical methods, without the prior written permission of the publisher, except in the case of brief quotations embodied in critical reviews and certain other noncommercial uses permitted by copyright law.

Table of Contents

Introduction – Aged 34 5

Introduction – Aged 21 7

Depression 8

    Physical Impact 9

    Brain Chemistry 9

    Stigma attached to Depression 10

    Types of Depression 10

    Treatments 11

    Outlook 11

How And Why Depression Occurs 13

What Depression Feels Like 17

    Self-Harm 21

    Fear of Dying 21

    Setback 23

Getting Through The Day 26

    Bedtime 31

    To Sum Up 33

An Example Of A Day In The Life Of A Seriously Depressed Person 34

Medical Help and Counselling 42

    Anti- Depressant Drugs 42

    How Anti-Depressant Drugs Work 42

    Different Types of Anti-Depressants 42

    How Anti-Depressants Effect You 42

    Counselling 43

Sorting Out Your Problems 44

Coping with Family, Friends and Events 49
    How to Cope with Friends, Family and Events 50
Eating Well and Exercise 53
Healing Through Self-Nurturance 56
Music & Writing 58
    Music 58
    Writing 58
Good Things That Come Out of Depression 60
Keeping Out of Depression 61

Introduction – Aged 34

At the age of 17, I started to feel unwell. I constantly felt sick and just wanted to be at home all the time. I went to the doctors on numerous occasions and finally, when I took my mum with me, the doctor told me I had depression and anxiety. He explained to me that depression was a chemical imbalance in the brain which was why I was feeling low. The reason I was feeling sick was because I was anxious. The doctor gave me some anti-depressants. I felt nervous about taking the tablets, but took them as I desperately wanted to feel well again.

It was a really tough time for me. My friends were doing their A-Levels and planning their university placements and I was stuck at home with nothing going on in my life. I had always wanted a career and presumed that I would be going to university, but I just didn't feel well enough.

I was referred to a counselling. Some of my sessions were funded by the NHS but I remember most of the sessions were funded by my parents. Looking back I don't know how they afforded this as we really didn't have any money. I started having acupuncture for my anxiety which helped me loads. Over time through the methods that I will share with you in this book, I started to feel better. Firstly I started noticing I had a whole day of feeling positive, then two days in a row, then a whole week and gradually over time I felt happy again. However, I still felt sick.

I went back to my doctors and said that I no longer felt depressed or anxious, but I still felt sick. The doctor ran some tests and it turned out that I had a stomach bug called Helicobacter Pylori, which causes stomach ulcers. That was why I had been feeling sick all this time!

After the treatment I felt much better. I started working part-time in a school as a classroom assistant and started a degree in Psychology with the Open University. Studying with the Open University meant I could study at home and still progress in my career like I wanted to. It actually meant that I paid for my course each year and had no living expenses because I was living at home with my mum (I completed my degree with no student debt). The degree helped me to get various full time posts such as a social work assistant in a medium secure unit and then as a counsellor.

I completed my psychology degree after 6 years. I decided to go to London and do a Masters degree in Business Psychology. I could never have imagined a few years back that I would be commuting to London to study for a Masters degree. After this I set up my own training and coaching company and have been running this for 7 years. I would have never have thought any of this was possible when I was younger and suffering with depression.

I wrote this book when I was 21 years old after recovering from my depression. It was published shortly afterwards thanks to funding from UnLtd, National Lottery. Unfortunately the publishers went bankrupt shortly afterwards. This year I found the manuscript and decided to self-publish it on Amazon. I have left the manuscript as it was, just tidying it up here and there to make sure it made sense. I wanted to keep it written by a young adult for teenagers and young adults. The introduction that follows is the introduction I wrote when I was 21 years old.

Introduction – Aged 21

Many young people are suffering from depression and anxiety in today's society. Young people often feel they are the only ones but there are literally thousands in the same position.

As you have already picked up this book, you are already on your way to recovery as you know or at least suspect there is a problem.

This book is not written by a person in the medical profession but by a person who has been through exactly the same as you, felt the same feelings, cried the same tears and like you will too, felt the elation of recovery.

Anybody can get better no matter who they are. Never give up and success will be yours.

I wish you all the luck in the future.

Depression

1 in 4 people will experience some kind of mental health problem in the course of a year (Mental Health Foundation 2014). Depression is one of the most common mental illnesses and tends to affect more women than men, especially when unemployed. Young people are at increasing risk as are very old people, particularly those who are ill or in pain.

Everybody feels down now and then. It could be a wide range of things that make them feel like this, such as Monday mornings, a row with the boss or partner, knocking a cup of tea over or even not being able to find their car keys. All of these little things tend to leave us feeling a bit low. Larger depressives may be financial difficulties, a relationship turning sour or your job being on the line. We also get depressed when friends or loved ones move or pass away. Feeling depressed is a natural part of life whether we like it or not.

The type of depression we are looking at in this book is long term depression, when you have felt really low for a lot more than just a couple of days or weeks. You may experience feelings of hopelessness, sadness or pessimism. Perhaps you have a lack of well-being and have begun to lose interest in your life altogether. You may experience moments of complete despair and find yourself bursting in to tears for no apparent reason. Your motivation levels could be at an all time low. You could be finding other people more irritating and intolerable. Perhaps you are experiencing feelings of guilt and thoughts of death may also be present.

The way you feel may vary throughout the day, some people feel better at the beginning of the day and some feel better at the end. As a depressive illness progresses the symptoms can become more intensified until the person gives up and spends most of their time in the comfort of their bed. This is only if they or everybody else fails to recognize the illness as depression.

Physical Impact

Depression not only impacts on your mind, it also impacts on your body. Symptoms range from insomnia and extreme lethargy to over-activeness. It can impact on appetite and weight gain. It can change your menstrual cycle and you may experience a lower sex drive. You might become more constipated. You may feel unexplained aches and pains. Whatever you experience you will tend to find your body and indeed your mind become tired very easily and your concentration span will probably be a lot shorter.

People who are depressed are often anxious too. When you are threatened you become anxious, even if the threat is in the imagination.

Anxiety can make you feel various physical symptoms such as nausea, dizziness, sweating, headaches and even muscular aches. These physical sensations, however horrible and terrifying they may be, CAN NOT ACTUALLY HARM YOU, they are harmless. So if you tend to feel sick when out, it can be quite comforting to know that the anxiety is very unlikely to make you sick, and as and when you return home these unpleasant feelings will disappear.

Brain Chemistry

Depression is often referred to as a chemical imbalance in the brain. There are various chemicals in the brain that are believed to play a role in depression. These chemicals are Acetylcholine, Serotonin, Norepinephrine, Dopamine, Glutamate and Gamma-aminobutyric acid. Serotonin, often called the 'happy chemical' impacts on mood. Research shows that people suffering with depression have reduced levels of serotonin. It is said Yoga encourages the body to produce more of this chemical, as does exercise.

Stigma attached to Depression

Unfortunately there can be a stigma attached to Depression. People can make assumptions and have little desire to learn about illnesses that do not concern them. They might believe they know how people get depression and never stop to listen to the real reasons behind depression. Some people may believe that negative, pessimistic people suffer with it and others don't. This is completely untrue ANYBODY CAN GET IT, AT ANYTIME IN THEIR LIVES. Some will read this and say 'Rubbish!' and they will think they are immune. Maybe even you thought like this yourself. Don't worry many of us have!

Fortunately depression is becoming less stigmatized and nowadays many more people understand the condition. It is now recognized as an illness and not as something that people 'bring upon themselves'. As a nation we are becoming better educated and more understanding.

Types of Depression

There are many different types of depression, most of which are mentioned below. It may be helpful, if you do not already know which type you are suffering from, to see if you recognize yourself in any of them.

Clinical Depression - this is the term given to people who are too depressed to help themselves and need expert assistance. The symptoms have persisted for more than a few weeks or months and interfere with work, family and social life.

Grief - Grief is a natural reaction to a loss. Those experiencing grief may also feel moments of happiness and are still looking forward to the future whereas someone with the medical condition of depression feels a lingering sadness. They find it difficult to enjoy anything and feel pessimistic about their future.

Postnatal Depression - after women have given birth some become low and depressed. Postnatal depression can start about six weeks after having a baby, but often it is not obvious until after 6 months. This may be due to the mother's hormones or of the reality of having a baby. It affects 1 in 10 new mothers. Symptoms include a feeling of not being able to cope, low mood and trouble sleeping.

S. A. D. - Seasonal Affective Disorder - triggered by the long hours of darkness during the winter months. Sufferers feel perfectly fine in the spring and summer, but become very depressed in the winter.

Treatments

The kind of treatment you need will depend on the type and severity of the illness. Counselling may be individual or group and you may need medication. For S.A.D., there are various methods to combat this type of depression, one being a light box. Your GP will discuss your treatment plan with you.

Outlook

The outlook is very bright for sufferers of depression. You stand a better chance of getting better if you speak with your GP and follow their advice.

If you think you have depression (it may help to read the chapter 'What Depression Feels Like' first) and have not yet visited your doctor it is very important that you do. If you are embarrassed you have no need to be. Your doctor sees people like you frequently and remember he has to deal with a lot more embarrassing ailments than depression!! So don't feel embarrassed. If you are uncomfortable about seeing a particular doctor as you believe he will be unsympathetic, arrange to see a different doctor.

I cannot stress enough how important it is to visit your GP if you think you are suffering with depressions. Your GP will know what treatment is best suited to your needs and prescribe it. Do not sit around telling yourself you will phone tomorrow or next week, phone now. If the surgery is not open read the rest of this section tomorrow morning. The longer you leave it the harder it is going to be. Do it now. Go on. Do just one positive thing today. Phone the doctors. Then you can reward yourself with a treat and give yourself a pat on the back. I realise this phone call will most likely take a lot of courage, but don't let your fear ruin your health. Go on, phone them. If you do it you'll feel a huge weight lifted from your shoulders. Some of you tough nuts won't find this a problem and deep down we all have the power to be tough nuts, right? So please phone today. Now in fact. Yes now!!

If your doctor does not take you seriously, then try again, do not give up. Try a different doctor, do anything to get heard. It is highly unlikely your doctor will not understand. If your GP does not take you seriously, then another GP will.

How And Why Depression Occurs

Frequently when people are suffering from depression there seems to be no single cause that stands out as to why they are feeling like this. It could have been triggered by hormonal disorders, medication, drugs or even physical illness. Brain chemistry can also play a part. Some types of depression run in families. It is possible to inherit a depressive illness. These are all biological reasons.

Depression may also occur due to social or psychological causes. Someone may undergo many changes or disturbing events thus causing mild to serious depression. They might be in an unhappy relationship or have severe financial problems, the list is endless.

Sometimes it can be tempting to ignore our problems and push them to the back our minds. Failing to face our problems can cause our mental health to suffer. We can hope that if we ignore them long enough they will get fed up and magically disappear. Sorry, but they probably won't. They will fester, damaging your mental health. Try to imagine a house in disrepair. If the owner doesn't do any maintenance or repairs, the house will finally rot and fall down. It is the same with your body. If you ignore your problems and leave them, your mental health will suffer and you may well find you have also 'fallen down'. It is up to us to help ourselves and do some repairs (see the chapter 'Sorting Out Your Problems'). The longer these problems are left not dealt with, the worse they seem to get until you believe they are not solvable. It is quite likely that you have read this section and think it does not apply to you because your problems are not solvable. I certainly used to think so. But however bad our problems seem there is more often than not a solution or at least ways to cope with them.

Maybe you have problems that upset you so much or are just too embarrassing to admit to. You have convinced yourself there is nothing wrong. In a way you have chosen to forget them as they hurt too much. This can be quite damaging. Now, I want you to take a moment to think about this. Go through your mind and ask yourself is there any problems you are trying to ignore? If you cannot think of any, then you have not got any. I do not want you to think some up or worrying that you can't find your problem. If you have a problem it will come clear in about 5 - 10 seconds. If your mind is a blank or many small problems pop into your head I want you to forget these for the moment. Just think about any serious problems you have not dealt with. By doing this you are being honest with yourself and realising you have a problem and it is not going to go away on its own accord. You do not need to think of solutions just yet (unless there is a time limit). We will work on it in the chapter 'Sorting Out Your Problems'. To sum up, not facing problems you know you have may lower your mood. It may just be a little dent in your overall happiness or it may be chronic.

Another factor which may lead to depression or certainly add to it is dreamlike ideas on how our life should be. Nearly everybody must have sat through an American sitcom and wish they had a life like theirs. A life that is full of fun and laughter 24 hours a day, lots of close pals, being extremely popular, all having boyfriends/girlfriends and to top it all off they are either filthy rich or stunningly beautiful. The thing you must realise is that it is fictional. It is made up and very, very few people have this cushy life-style. Yes it would be great and life is often like this, just not constantly.

But have you ever noticed they never laugh at each other? Only the audience laughs. It is probable that if someone was to record your life for the day it would be just as funny. It's watching others that is often the funny part. However sometimes these programmes can leave us feeling jealous and depressed that our lives are not this much fun and we want them to be. When the actors are interviewed they often comment they wish their life was as perfect as their characters.

Life is also not like English soaps, thankfully. The soaps only tend to get really good ratings when there is a drama such as a court case, murder, kidnapping, stabbing etc. These dramatic events attract the most viewers. So when we watch these soaps there is hardly ever anything nice happening. We watch these soaps and think life is like this. People barely ever laugh or have fun. So we have this depressed outlook on life and many people become paranoid they'll have the same misfortunes as the people they see on television. Honestly if we had all the bad luck they have in one street, we would move away! How can one street have so many disasters? At least life is not like this.

So here we have two extremes. One being fantastic and the other being dreadful! Life truly is somewhere in the middle and varies in both directions.

Another thing a lot of people find depressing is the news. The only news reported is bad news, so again we think life is full of crime. I certainly thought so until a close friend pointed out there is more good news than bad. However, the news broadcasters do not consider good news as important, so they do not bother to report it. Overall life is a lot better than we see it on television. The shows get better viewings if they are dramatic and they do not bother to report good news. It's no wonder so many people get depressed!

Another aspect which may contribute to your depression is how sadness is often considered a bad thing. For example, if you are at college/work and in a terrible mood, people tend to take it personally or mock you for being a grumpy person! This in turn can put you in an even worse mood. Also in some TV shows people are very rarely sad. Therefore we may perceive sadness shouldn't happen. Many of us have the misconception that we always have to be happy and you should 'live life to the max', 'don't worry, be happy', 'unhappiness is an unnatural state'. All of these slogans tell us we should be ecstatically happy and should count our blessings. Unfortunately it is not easy being happy all the time, so when we do feel sad we may put a front on and pretend we are happy. We might try to fake our happiness so we do not get thought of as a grumpy, moody person. Sometimes we disallow our negative emotions without even realising we are doing it. By not admitting our negative feelings and hiding them away, we can project them on to others. We take it out on them.

Another aspect of living that can make people feel down at times is the feeling that life is mundane. Life, at times, can seem to get a bit boring. One thing you could do though if you have got the urge to try something different is to try a new activity. Take up a new hobby that you enjoy such as learning to play a musical instrument. Perhaps you could do a bungee jump or a parachute jump for charity. The list is endless.

To be happy all the time is a tremendous pressure. Often deep down we are hurting and have no one to talk to. We may feel we don't want to damage our reputation of being 'happy go lucky' and carefree. As said previously not talking about problems tends to make them seem a lot worse. Talking about problems helps a lot more than you think. If you have no one to confide in, then you can call a designated helpline. A simple web search can help you find designated help-lines or you can ask your GP.

Negative emotions are not bad things. They are natural and useful. Negative emotions often tell us that something is wrong and we need to take action.

So from this chapter you may have realised a few things which have contributed towards your depression. Alternatively, there may be one thing which you know has caused it such as a relationship breakdown or suffering with ill health. It is natural to feel upset with such events, and it would be odd if we did not feel depressed. You may have had mild depression and this devastating shock was just too much for you to cope with, so you fell into a deeper depression. Hopefully by now most of you know, or at least suspect, what has contributed to your depression. For some of you, you may still be in the dark as to why you feel this way. A counsellor may be helpful here. Whatever your case we are going to get you well, you CAN beat it. If I can beat depression, anyone can. With the help of this book we are going to get you fighting fit. One of the most important things that I cannot stress enough is however hard it gets, however sad you feel, NEVER EVER GIVE UP.

What Depression Feels Like

Sometimes people don't realise they have depression. They may have had it a few years, steadily feeling worse until it finally gets to the point where they feel they cannot go on and life has little meaning. Even at this point they can fail to realise they have depression until it is pointed out to them or they read an article that rings true for them.

When I was unaware I had depression, I read a six page article on Depression. It still did not click! I just thought I was a gloomy person and it was my fault I felt like this. Anything that promised happiness or had the word happiness in the title I would have to have.

At least you know or at least suspect you have Depression. This is one of the biggest steps to recovery, knowing you have a problem. So well done! It is a bit like alcoholics. They do not think they have a problem but as soon as they realise they do, they can start to get better.

To a depressed person life may seem pointless and boring. The world seems a horrible place to be, full of crime, murder, famine and hate. You may focus on bad things like illness and world disasters and completely disregard many good things. You may feel as though there is little or no point in struggling through every minute of torture. Recovery is hard but the rewards are endless and are definitely worth the effort. It may not seem like it to you right now, but it will get better and you will find life easier. Anyone who has recovered from depression will tell you this.

I know you may feel like giving up. You may have had thoughts of committing suicide but I can give you many reasons why you should never, however bad things get, do this. Some of the main reasons are listed below. If you are feeling suicidal please phone your GP or contact your hospital immediately.

1. IT IS PERMANENT - however long recovery takes you will still have the rest of your life to live and to enjoy. You will probably be happier than ever before due to your experiences.

2. YOU NEVER KNOW WHAT IS JUST AROUND THE CORNER. For all you know you could win the lottery tomorrow or a competition. You could fall in love or have a whirlwind romance. I know you may think none of this will ever happen to you, but how do you know?

3. THINK OF THOSE YOU WOULD LEAVE BEHIND. However much you hurt now, your closest relatives and friends are going to hurt so much if you take your life. Do you really want to inflict that pain on people who love you and who you love? You may have the excuse 'But nobody would miss me.' This is complete and utter rubbish. When you have depression you probably have this thought fairly often, because you feel unloved and think everybody is sick of you. I certainly did. But people do love you even if they might not show it every day. They would be devastated if they lost you. They would be devastated even if they knew you were contemplating killing yourself. These people need you as much as you need them.

4. THINGS WILL GET BETTER. To be honest you are probably lower than low and it couldn't be much worse, so looking on the bright side things can only get better can't they? The only way is up. You have hit the bottom and are now going to propel yourself all the way to the top.

When I was very low I felt like hibernating. This was not a reasonable solution to coping with depression, especially because in the end it would be so boring!

So to sum up the way to beat depression is to work on your recovery. You need to try your best to get well if not for you, then for your family and friends (this is what kept me going).

Everybody's experience of depression is different. Everybody experiences different sensations, thoughts and feelings. I will describe how I and other sufferers have felt while going through depression. You may have some or nearly all of the feelings that will be mentioned. This is again another important stage in your recovery, as you realise your thoughts and feelings are perfectly natural when going through depression and you are not alone. By knowing a lot of people have felt like you do now and are now completely well you can feel confident that you too can feel better. Depression is described by many people as feeling as though you are in a very deep black hole and you are completely surrounded by darkness. Some people describe it as a feeling of isolation, whilst other people feel suffocated and slightly warm. Whatever you feel, one thing is for sure it is almost unbearable. You don't know where to put yourself or what to do. You manage to take a few steps forward only to take a few steps back again. Once this keeps happening there seems little point in trying again, but you must. By all means take a break but NEVER give up.

You may find part of you indulges in your sadness. Perhaps a small part of you doesn't want to try to get better. It seems like an effort to even get up and make a drink let alone begin the task of climbing out of your depression. You can feel like you just can't be bothered. I do not blame you for this. It is exactly how I felt. Some of you reading this may have already overcome this stage, if so well done. If not, it is not a problem as this will be your next aim and I will guide you as to how to get the motivation you need.

Depression is extremely emotionally painful at times and you may be surprised that you can even feel as low as you do. You feel alone and isolated. Even if you have company, you still may feel alone and cut off from the world. It is as if life is not happening. It is as if you are not really there. The term used for this is 'alienation'.

It appears that nobody understands you. You many think that nobody knows what you are going through, how you are feeling or how hard it is for you. It makes everything seem harder to do and seem less worthwhile. Seeing friends and even family takes a huge amount of effort and courage as you try to put on a 'happy face' and make conversation. You may start to dread their calls. You can feel like you want to cut yourself off from others to avoid the bother.

Sometimes you will want and need to be on your own. Other times you do not want to be on your own but you may feel like you do not want to be with anyone either. In this case it would be a good idea to use the phone or text. It is important to see people if only occasionally. It may feel a bit like a duty but so be it, otherwise when you are fit and happy you may well be friendless and we do not want that do we?

You may see others smiling, laughing, joking and believe they are faking it. This could be because at times you know that you fake it. In this world, others' lives can look so much fun, but you never know what is going on under the surface. People can filter their lives so you only see the positive aspects.

There are literally thousands of people who are going through exactly what you are. There are also literally thousands of people who have been through it and can now say 'I used to be like you and now look at me! I've never been happier with my life.' You might think 'Well bully for you! Yeah you can do it, but I'm not you. You couldn't have felt as bad as I do because I know I can't do it.' But you can. You will. If you suffer from an anxiety disorder this may be particularly hard to imagine, but trust me it is possible. I know it does not feel that way right now, but it is.

When I was in the depths of my depression I was extremely confused, my head was a jumble of messed up thoughts, I spent countless hours trying to work out how to make my life better, how to be happier, nicer to know etc. Yet I hardly ever came up with anything and if I did it would not be long before I discarded my thoughts. When you are suffering with depression you might find that your concentration span is extremely short. I found most things dead boring (except television). Nothing satisfied me so I got agitated. Sometimes I would feel so agitated that I would injure myself by biting something really hard until my jaw hurt or kicking something and nearly breaking my foot. This may sound strange to some of you, but I got my frustration with myself out of me. This is sometimes labelled as self-harm.

Self-Harm

Self-harm is a lot more common than we are lead to believe. Literally thousands of young people inflict violence upon themselves every day. It can range from cigarette burns, pinching and biting themselves to banging their heads against the wall and even using razors to cut themselves. The person who self-harms may feel addicted to it. It is something they feel compelled to do. In a way it is their crutch, a way to cope with their life. Self-harm can affect anyone at any age.

What leads people to this devastating act? Sometimes the person is feeling emotional pain and to stop themselves emotionally hurting they harm themselves. They then feel the physical pain and their emotional pain is blocked out. Some people who self-harm do it because they feel they need to be punished. Others feel frustrated with themselves or stressed. Self-harm can become a habit. If the person is considered to be a threat to their own safety, they are likely to be referred to a specialist unit where they are kept under supervision and treated. If you are self-harming you can go to your GP for help, or call the Samaritans or MIND. You can find their telephone numbers online. There is also a great website www.selfharm.co.uk which you may find helpful. It might be a case of finding a more positive outlet for your emotions. A friend of mine who suffered seriously from self-harm said, 'It is a way of getting your hurt out and away from you, it is a way of expressing yourself. Now I write poems which has exactly the same effect.'

Fear of Dying

Another common feeling people experience is that of the fear of dying. Many (I certainly was) are basically convinced they are going to die. Every headache, stomach ache or any other ailment they experience is considered serious. Some people will go to the doctors every week whilst others will suffer in silence. The important thing to remember here is that it is a natural part of depression. As depression lessens so will your fears. I know this is probably of no comfort to you right now. It can be extremely frightening thinking you are seriously ill. It can be draining thinking that your really bad headache means that you have a brain tumour. During depression your immune system is likely to be fairly low so you may find yourself frequently feeling under the weather. Also stress causes headaches, muscle aches, eating problems and so on. If it makes you feel better to go to the doctors, then do so. If you are worried about a long-standing ailment, your mind will be put at rest or the problem will be addressed.

You may be worried about going into hospital. I do not think there are many people in this world who are not. If it happens, it happens. You would cope. You would get through it. I know you might feel scared but you would be in the good hands of the medical team.

If you do know of health problems such as a dodgy heart, asthma etc. and you feel a bit strange in that aspect do not hesitate to get in contact with someone from the medical profession.

Below is a list of other feelings/thoughts and physical effects of depression you may experience.

You may feel nothing and nobody can help.

You feel you will be like this all your life.

Your head is a jumble of thoughts. (To sort this out see the chapter 'Sorting Out Your Problems'.)

Dislike/hate yourself.

Dislike/hate people in general.

Few positive thoughts, many negative thoughts.

Feel numb, empty, despondent.

Blaming yourself and feeling unnecessarily guilty about things.

Big effort to do the smallest of things.

Cannot make decisions.

Difficulty in sleeping or staying asleep.

Loss of appetite.

Eating more. Eating less. Eating lots of unhealthy foods.

Use tobacco, alcohol and other drugs a lot more.

Short concentration span, everything boring and short lived. Nothing satisfies. Easily agitated.

Bleak outlook on life and the world.

Confused easily.

May feel ugly and fat etc.

Feel, 'No one has the right to be happy because the world is so horrible.'

Wishing you had never been born.

Wanting to save others from this horrible world.

Harrowing thoughts. For example fearing for others safety when they go out of the house or are late to return.

You may also get depressed that you have depression. This in turn adds to your depression. Many people feel depressed that they are depressed. This element of depression can feel more intense than the original depression.

Setback

Setback can be devastating. You think you are getting somewhere, you have felt happier than you can remember for a long time, the world is not quite as bad as you thought, the sun is out and you feel fantastic. Or perhaps you are just getting those first glimpses of life after depression and feel excited about your future. Then all of a sudden, your world comes crashing down around your ears again. You might think, 'Why do I bother?' Well the answer is that you bother because you are a very brave, intelligent and courageous person. Everybody experiences various setbacks, but you must accept this. When you experience a setback, look at it as a break. You are working really hard and are making great steps to feeling happy again. Take off two days if you can and do whatever you like. Spoil yourself rotten. But do not indulge in self-pity. After your rest you will be spilling over with energy and you will have regained your courage, spirit and enthusiasm to go on to the next stage.

This diagram shows setback and the upward trend towards recovery.

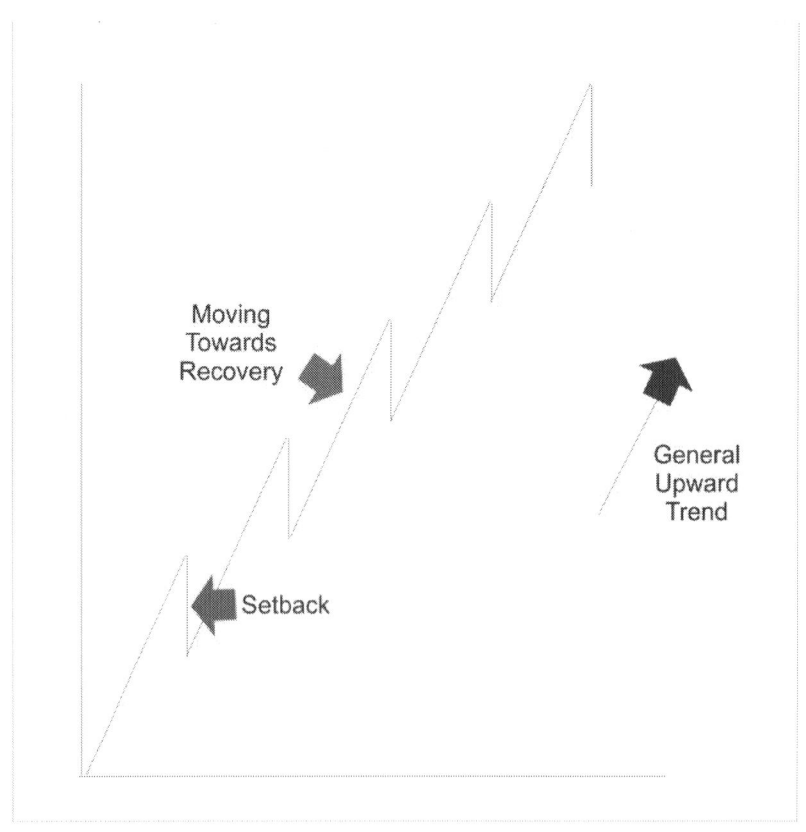

The general trend is upwards. So even if you feel you are back to where you started, think again! You are not. Take a break for your good efforts!

Getting Through The Day

You wake and for a split second you feel good and glad to be alive. You are looking forward to your day. Then ye-ouch! It dawns on you that you might struggle to get through the day. Okay, you got through yesterday so what's so different about today? You might feel like you can't face it. Perhaps your mind fills with despair, your pulse races and you feel anxious. You might decide you don't want to get up and at the same time you don't want to stay in bed. You feel you need someone to help you but there are lots of things you can do to help yourself. In this chapter we will look at making the days a bit more bearable. Unfortunately, I cannot take all the pain away as that will only happen in time. But I can certainly lessen it.

First of all we need to start the day as we mean to go on. As soon as you wake up tomorrow the first thing I want you to do is jump, yes JUMP up and open your curtains. Then open the window and breathe in some fresh air. This will make you feel good. Okay, the next step is to get dressed. It is best to do this before breakfast when you are suffering with depression because after breakfast it will hang over you like a dark cloud. You may feel drained and like you can't be bothered to get dressed and then slob around in your nightwear watching television and feel down. We do not want this. We want you up and dressed and feeling good. You can have a shower if you like or if you do not feel up to it, have a bath. It is important you have a wash every day to keep you feeling fresh as feeling fresh promotes good feelings.

Okay, so now we are up and dressed and feeling better than yesterday. You may feel a bit tired but this is understandable as depression can make you feel tired. Next on our list is breakfast and for those of you who skip it please try eating something. Some people find breakfast a whole task in itself. The anxious feelings you get can make it an extreme chore, so we need to change this. We need something that you enjoy such as some nice fruit, a boiled egg or a bacon sandwich that you can eat on the days you find eating breakfast difficult.

How you cope with your day depends on what you do. There are different circumstances for different people. This next section is for people who have to go to work, college or school. Even if you do not it may be interesting for you to read.

One of the hardest things about going to work/college or school is not feeling up to going. If you have days like this then it is important that you talk to the manager or the head teacher. If you are at school and you do not feel up to going in every single day of the week then you must go and see your head teacher. If possible talk to your parents and ask them to come with you. If they do not understand then take a close friend. If there is no one, then go on your own. It is important that you do go, as it takes off the pressure, which will help to relieve your depression. One of the hardest things about both depression and anxiety is explaining your illness to others. As it is a psychological illness people cannot see it so they may not believe it exists. Therefore it is necessary to map out what you are going to say. Tell them you are suffering from depression and anxiety (if this is so) and it produces physical symptoms so sometimes you feel you are unable to stay at work/college or school for the whole day. If at school you could ask if you could take your work home with you or take some time off.

If you are at work and struggling to cope, then it would be a good idea to speak to your GP. They may provide you with a medical certificate. Tell your employer that you are depressed and find it difficult to complete your work tasks some days. Maybe you could work from home, cut your hours, only work once or twice a week or go off sick for a period of time.

If your head teacher or manager refuses to listen, then do not despair. We can still get you through this. If you are at college you could take a year out. If you are at work consider leaving and then re-applying somewhere else. I know this is not the ideal situation but sometimes we do not have a choice. If you decide to stay at work or college then try to follow this simple guide.

1. Get early nights.

2. Do exercise (see the chapter 'Eating Well and Exercise'). You may not feel like it sometimes, which is fine.

3. Eat healthily. The most important thing right now is your health.

If you are at home all day:

Now to people who work or study this sounds ideal. Yes it is better than going to work as it takes the pressure off but it can still be difficult.

You might feel like you have nothing to do all day and are not sure how to fill your hours. On the other-hand you might also feel like you have so many chores to do that you feel overwhelmed. You may find it difficult to know where to start and wonder where you are going to find the energy. You are shattered and exhausted yet you have done nothing. You can feel frustrated as you are bored and want to do something, yet everything is such an effort.

Boredom is a terrible thing. It can make you feel really down. Unfortunately it also gives you time to dwell on your problems and circumstances. Always remember an active mind is a happy mind.

So our main aims are to keep you active thus producing positive emotions. By active I do not mean jumping up and down, never stopping. I just mean keeping your MIND active. If your mind is full of activity then there is very little room for depressive, negative thoughts to creep in. We need to make a list of the things you enjoy which you feel capable of doing.

Activities could include:

Friends you could see during the day.
Bike ride
Computer games
Going to the shops and buying a magazine
Exercise
Cooking

Drawing

Walking

Learn a new skill e.g. musical instrument, how to apply make-up, how to become a writer etc.

Make your list as long as you possibly can even if the things you write down seem boring and something you would never usually do such as weeding.

Write down everything you can think of doing and I want you to try everything at least once on this list in the next two months if possible. Going back to the title of this chapter, 'Getting through the day' I have drawn out a time plan for your day - trying to make it as easy as possible for you. You do not have to stick to it at all. Feel free to change it, add to it, lessen it, do whatever you like, it is only a rough idea.

8am. Wake up. Jump out of bed. Open curtains. Open window. Deep breaths of fresh air.

8.05am. Take a bath, shower or have a wash.

8.20am. Have a big gorgeous breakfast. Enjoy a piece of fruit. Watch television or listen to the radio. Do not sit on your own in the quiet, as this is a perfect moment for nasty thoughts to creep in to your mind about the day ahead. Have a little rest.

Go to Work, College or School. (If you still have to.)

If you are at home:

9am. Now is the time to do any housework. You may feel like saving it for later on in the day as something to do but it will only hang over you and make you feel depressed. So do it now.

9.45am. Rest time. Watch television, listen to the radio or read a book.

10.30am. Now if you feel up to it go out even if it is just for a walk or to see a friend. If you do not feel up to it and it is warm enough then sit or walk in the garden. If it is raining or too cold outside do something constructive indoors. You could rearrange your room, design new colours for it, bake a cake or do some drawing. Even if you don't feel up to doing anything, try to do something. Remember an active mind is a happy mind. Even if it is something you find boring, just try it.

12.30pm. Okay. It is dinnertime. For many people this is just as hard as breakfast. Try to eat, even if just a little.

1pm. Well done! You are basically half way through. We are getting there! You could watch television now or read a book. Give yourself a break.

2pm. Now look at your list of things to do. Is there anything you fancy doing? Try a couple of things.

3. 30pm. Time to go out again for a walk or go on your bike. If you do not feel up to it you could try some gentle exercise at home maybe just dance round your room. You may feel stupid but no one can see you if the curtains are shut! Doing exercise at this time of day breaks up the day and increases positive feelings. It leaves you feeling active which is good for the evening.

4. 15pm. Rest.

4.30pm. Decide now what you want for dinner. You can prepare it now so it's all ready. Then take some time to relax. It is important you rest during depression as it is a very exhausting emotion.

Come home from work, college or school.

Next:

5. 30pm. Eat dinner. If you are on your own and feel lonely have the radio or the television on. The reason I suggest watching the television or having the radio on is that they are a good source of human company and can be very comforting when you feel lonely.

6pm. Let your dinner go down.

6. 30pm. Wash up.

7pm. If you can, phone up a friend or relative and invite them around. I know it seems a huge effort but once you see them you will forget your problems and feel better. If you really do not want to see anyone, then it is important we have something that will occupy you for the evening, maybe hire a video or plan a lovely night in.

Whatever you do try not to dwell on tomorrow too much and if you do, think of something you would like to do. Remember the thought of the next day is often a lot worse in your mind than it is in reality.

You can frequently take comfort in the thought that you are not alone. There are thousands of people exactly like you, in your situation and experiencing the same feelings as you do day in, day out.

Bedtime

For some bedtime is the end of an exhausting, painful day. A time when they can relax and finally be at ease but for others it is yet again another challenge, a task that fills them with dread and turmoil. If you are one of these people, do not despair we are helping you now. Many people suffering from depression suffer from insomnia. It can be so frustrating, you feel tired, yet you cannot sleep. You feel wide awake but too tired to get up. In this section we will look at ways in which we can help you sleep and how to cope if you wake in the night.

First of all one thing you must realise is rest is very close to the sleep state. Lying down and closing your eyes is nearly as good as sleep itself. So if you cannot sleep bear this thought in mind and it should be of some comfort to you that you are still reviving your body and gaining energy for the next day. Do not get into the pattern of thinking, 'I do not want to go to bed as there is no point because I will not sleep anyway.' If you constantly think you will not be able to sleep, then you will not, whereas if you try and discard all your bad nights and start afresh each night you have a better chance of sleeping. Each night before you go to bed, picture yourself succeeding, picture yourself falling asleep. Your mind will try to follow what it pictures.

Now to increase your chances of sleeping even more, we need to prepare. The idea is that you start to relax before you even contemplate going to bed. You can start however early in the evening you like. Some people believe watching television is relaxing but various studies have shown this is not true. Yes, you are resting your body and this is good but you are not relaxing your mind. There is a difference. So we need to find activities that relax you, maybe one of the following activities will help.

1. Take a bath. Use relaxing oil or bath foam if possible. Perhaps you could light some candles.

2. Go to your bedroom. Dim the lights or use candles and listen to relaxing music.

3. Read a book.

4. Listen to an audio book. Many libraries now have free audio books as part of their lending service. You can often download them to your phone for free via an app.

Before you go to bed some people find a warm milky drink relaxing and comforting. There are a few you can try such as cocoa; malt drinks, milky decaffeinated tea or some prefer just plain milk.

It is better to get ready for bed before you start your relaxing methods as getting changed makes your body active and puts all that relaxation straight down the drain.

Once you are fully relaxed you can get in to bed, maybe read for a little while to make you really tired. Then switch off your bedside light and you will fall into a deep, deep sleep.

What happens if you cannot sleep? First of all try this simple trick. A lot of the time the reason you cannot sleep is because you keep twisting and turning. So look at your clock and say to yourself 'I am going to stay in one position for 10 minutes with my eyes shut.' By the end of the 10 minutes you will either be asleep or very drowsy. If you are drowsy do another 10 minutes. If you move before the 10 minutes is up, then start the 10 minutes again.

If this does not work then get up. This breaks the pattern of not sleeping. Aim to stay up for 15 minutes. You can read, have a quick bath, go for a walk around the house, make another milky drink or anything else you would like to do. Then go back to bed. Lay still with your eyes closed for 10 minutes. Try to physically relax your muscles in your body. Do not try to force the sleep.

If the reason you cannot sleep is for problems milling around in your head, then write down all your problems and thoughts as if you were telling a friend. If you feel lonely put the television or radio on low and leave it on while you fall asleep.

To Sum Up

Throughout the day you may get various feelings. Some will be good, some will be bad. Once we know what they are they become easier to deal. We begin to accept them as part of depression. Just try to bide your time and understand that the feelings you are experiencing are a symptom of your illness. There are thousands of people going through exactly the same and you WILL get through them.

An Example Of A Day In The Life Of A Seriously Depressed Person

Monica is 20. She lives in a semi-detached house with her Mum, Dad and two sisters. She has a part time job in a local bakery. Monica has quite a few good friends and a boyfriend who is called Matt. They have been together for four months. (This story is loosely based on me.)

'I wake up in the mornings usually at about nine. I could easily sleep for longer but I have to start work at ten. The split second I wake up I feel pretty well, then it gradually worsens and by the time I get up I feel worse than before I went to bed. Often in the mornings when I sit up I have a huge dizzy spell and panic. I feel I won't be well enough to go to work and I worry I'll get the sack. But as a rule it always passes (1). I go downstairs. I'm usually on my own at this time as everybody has gone to work or school. So instead of sitting up at the table, I eat my cornflakes in front of the television. I don't really enjoy breakfast T.V. but it is company (2). In fact it bores me but I cannot bear to be on my own as I just feel so much hurt. I did try the radio but nah T.V. is the best for me as I can actually see the people. Once I can gather enough energy, I usually have a shower (3). I stand up in the shower just wishing I could flop down into the corner and sit there for a few minutes (4). I get dressed for work and have the same 'morning argument' with myself. It goes something like this:

"Shall I go to work?"
"Yes."
"But do I feel up to it?"
"Yes you do."
"No, I am going to be ill. I actually feel ill today. What if I go to work and I can't cope. How will I explain to the boss that I don't feel well enough to finish my shift?"
"You will not be ill."

This drives me mad. I read once that when you have depression or anxiety these 'two people' in your head are actually quite common. This is reassuring for me as I worried about this. (5).

After this argument with myself I usually try and force myself to go as I am always alright. Sometimes I don't go and when I don't I feel awful for the rest of the day. I constantly think I'd be nearly home now and I kick myself. It's a horrible feeling, as I just do not know where to turn (6). I only work for 4 hours but that is enough. It amazes me how people can work all day. Why don't they feel bad like I do? I know some do (7). But I'm talking about well people. Why aren't they sad like me?

I go to work on the bus. It's not far to work, only five minutes on the bus. I find the bus a challenge as well (8). The bus is very crowded in the mornings. I sit on my own praying nobody will sit next to me or talk to me or know me! I know this must sound horrible but I'm in a world of my own and I don't want anyone to invade my space. One morning I sat there and a man sat next to me who smelt of last night's curry. Urgh! It made me feel so ill.

I arrive at work by 10 am, put my coat downstairs and get changed. I have to put an act on now to be happy and smiley to everyone, sometimes I just wish I could just stick my tongue out! (9). I look at the food and my stomach turns. How will I get through the day? And how will I eat lunch?

A customer comes in and I serve him. He takes my mind off being ill especially as he is good looking! But as if he would fancy me, I'm ugly (10). My boyfriend says I'm pretty but he must be blind. I don't know why he goes out with me really. I'm horrible to him and he just puts up with it. I kick myself sometimes, I so much want to be nice but I just go in a grump, get attention and don't want to lose it (11).

The first half an hour at work goes pretty fast as we are quite busy (12) at this time. When it slows down a bit at about 10.45am, that's usually when I think I've got ages to go. I usually have a little panic attack now and have to go downstairs to sort myself out (13). The things that mill around in my head are mainly, 'I cannot cope. I do not know why I bother coming to work. I'm going to give it up. Oh! I feel ill. Somebody help me.' I've usually been in the loo for five minutes by now so I have to force myself out and go back upstairs. But boy! Is it hard! I wish I could stay in the toilet all day!

We have an early lunch at 11.30am because of the lunchtime rush. I'm not usually hungry at this time (14), but I have to eat otherwise I would be hungry later and feel ill. I have a roll, a packet of crisps and a cup of tea. As I'm eating I usually have the boss hanging over me trying to be pleasant but sometimes I just wish I was just left alone. I really don't like people watching me eat. I also feel pressured to keep eating, even if I don't want to (15).

After eating lunch I feel a huge relief, but unfortunately it is now time to clean the bakery machines which I dislike doing as they smell awful. I tell myself I can handle it because I know I can, though it is hard. I always manage to do it, even if it means clenching my jaw and holding my breath (16). Once that is over I know the day is on its way out. By now it is usually about 12.15pm and the lunchtime rush starts. I don't get time to think about my problems - which is good (17). I sometimes get panicked when I look at what I am doing, all those people, but I cope.

At about 1.45pm it tends to quieten down. I usually panic now as I have nothing to do except think. But then I realise its only 15 minutes to go and that makes me feel better. 2 o'clock comes and I can go home. At last I walk out of the bakery and I am so happy. I did it! Unfortunately this happiness doesn't tend to last as I think of what is to come such as waiting for a bus, doing the housework chores, including cooking dinner, and then getting through the evening. It's as if everything I do in my life is a task (18). I may enjoy it when I'm there but the thought of seeing my friend tonight and trying to be happy is such an effort. I feel like cancelling and having an easy night in with my boyfriend, but I want to see my friend.

Anyway, the bus journey home goes okay, I'm usually starving so tend to feel a bit sick but I know it is hunger. I get home and just slump in the chair absolutely exhausted but don't know why (19). I've only worked 4 hours. I used to do 9 hours! I feel hurt, lonely and bored (20). I look at the mountain of washing up (21), and put the telly on instead. I usually watch it for an hour while eating junk food (22). Then I start on the housework. I feel annoyed at having to do it. I usually feel very depressed at this time of day (23). I don't know why, but it is as regular as clockwork.

My sisters get home from school/college and I hibernate in my bedroom (24). I cannot bear to socialise especially not today when I've got my friend coming around tonight. The phone often rings and I dread to think it is for me. When it is I sometimes pretend that I'm not here because I can't be doing with it (25). Mum and Dad both work so I prepare the dinner. I hate doing this. It puts a dampener on the day. I don't know why but is such an effort.

Next Mum and Dad get home. I hate this time of day. The house gets so noisy. I know I must sound like an old fogey but I don't care.

We eat dinner together which I find a huge challenge. Sitting up at the table with everyone I feel like I'm on show. I hate it (26).

Afterwards, whatever I have planned for the evening I debate whether I feel up to it. The depressive feelings usually kick in now, big time. I just want to hibernate, shut myself away and never talk to anyone ever again. I get a pain in my stomach (27).

Friends usually come around at about seven. I know this sounds horrible but I usually can't wait for them to go (28). It's not that I don't like them, far from it, they're great! It's not that I don't want to see them either. I just can't be bothered because I am just so exhausted I just want to be with my family, with my boyfriend or on my own. When I am with my friends I am usually okay and do feel better as I forget my problems and they make me laugh (29). But I sometimes I fake my laughter and pretend to be happy (30). I just don't have as much fun as I used to (31). They seem to have such good lives full of fun, blokes and going out. It makes me so jealous. They never seem to be sad. Whenever you speak to them they are happy, bubbly and full of energy (32). So why am I dull, depressed and *only have enough energy to fuel an ant? (33). When my friends come round we normally stay in as that is all I feel up to. If we do go out I'm usually fine actually, as I suppose I put on a brave act again.*

Anyway, they usually go pretty early, I don't know why. Maybe it's because they find me boring (34). I'm scared to lose my friends because of my depression. When they go, I go straight to bed and normally feel very depressed about my life (35). I watch television. It usually takes me 2-3hrs to get to sleep. I don't often wake during the night, but if I do it fills me with panic (36) and I feel really depressed when I start to think about things happening in my life (37). I often cry myself to sleep in a state of despair (38).'

If you match the numbers in the section above to the numbers below you will see why Monica was feeling like she was and how she can help herself.

1. The reason for the dizzy spell is she is probably getting up too quickly. When you have depression you have to be gentle with yourself and do things slowly. Her immediate reaction is to panic. She has no reason to panic. If she reassures herself it is only because she has got up too quick she will no longer panic. You may feel a bit ill in the mornings but I assure you these feelings will pass quickly.

2. This is very good. Television can be great company and takes your mind off your problems and some of the hurt you feel.

3. She should have had a shower as soon as she got up because now, after breakfast, she feels lethargic.

4. Depression is exhausting and even showering can seem like a huge effort. The thought of the day ahead may leave you just wanting to sit down and avoid getting on with what you need to do.

5. Monica is correct. It is very common to have 'two voices' that argue inside your head. Most people have these two voices even if they have not suffered from mental health issues. Try to let the positive one win.

Encourage it. Remember it is very common and you are perfectly normal. When your depression subsides you will find these voices will lessen too. Try to lighten the situation up by painting images in your head of what the two people look like.

6. Often in depression you will experience the feeling of not knowing where to turn. It is horrible and I am afraid you just have to bide your time. It will pass fairly quickly.

7. They don't feel bad like you because they have not got depression. Depression is exhausting.

8. If you have problems going on a bus, think of it as a big car. Try listening to music on your headphones to keep yourself calm.

9. Putting on an act can be draining.

10. When you are depressed you may have very little self-esteem so you may feel ugly, fat etc. This is not true. It is just low self-esteem.

11. When you are depressed you feel like you want some comfort and love from someone. When you are feeling good they think you don't need it, but you still do. If you feel positive, show it and get positive attention that way.

12. If you keep busy you will feel better.

13. It would have been better if she had stayed put and engaged herself in an activity.

14. As Monica is not that hungry she could eat half and save half for later.

15. She could pretend to put the food down because she was talking and concentrating on that.

16. Clenching your teeth is the worst thing to do. Try and relax your body and you will find you feel better.

17. Keeping your mind active will help you to not think about your problems for a while.

18. When you are depressed everything can feel like an effort.

19. Working whilst suffering with depression can really deplete your energy leaving you feeling exhausted even after a relatively short shift.

20. Feeling lonely, hurt and bored are common feelings of depression. Try to accept it.

21. Monica could have done the washing up before she left if she felt up to it. She finds out it is a depressing thing to come home to.

22. Eating junk food can make you feel worse about yourself if you are watching your diet or your health.

23. This is understandable. Monica bas been to work, she then sits in front of the television eating junk foods and knowing she has some chores to do. It would be best if she had a 20 minute rest, did the housework and then have something healthier to eat. Then she can sit down and rest.

24. Wanting to hibernate is a part of depression. People often find they don't want to be on their own either.

25. Here she is using avoiding tactics to make herself feel better. It is okay to do this sometimes but do not do it all the time as it becomes a habit and you may lose all your friends.

26. Being 'on show' when you feel low is awful. However, socialising and receiving the support of your family can help a great deal.

27. You may experience physical symptoms during depression.

28. Monica is just tired. Socialising can be a real effort when you are suffering with depression. It is nothing to feel bad about.

29. Good therapy! Forgetting your problems for a while is what we want.

30. Hopefully your friends will understand your illness so you won't have to fake your happiness.

31. Because she is depressed, she is ill, she was not before.

32. You never really know what other people's lives are like until you are them. People often filter their lives, so you only see the positive elements. It's human nature. They want to impress others. On their own or with their family they may be very different people.

33. Because she is ill and as mentioned earlier it is exhausting.

34. Monica is not boring, just a little low.

35. Other people's lives always seem much better than our own. As they say, 'The grass is always greener on the other side.' If you were them you would realise their lives are not perfect either and you may even be jealous of yourself.

36. Waking in the night can make you panic. Try to relax, listen to some relaxing music, read a book or have a milky drink.

37. Things always seem worse at night time because you are tired. Things will look a lot rosier in the morning.

38. You can gain a lot of comfort from crying as long as you don't let it get hysterical. Crying can help to relieve the pressure.

Medical Help and Counselling

There are three ways you can help yourself to recovery, these are medication, counselling and self-help books such as this one. For your best chances of recovery a combination of all three is recommended.

Anti- Depressant Drugs

Doctors do not usually prescribe these drugs to people with a minor depressive illness, such as a short term problem where the emotional pain will soon pass. One example would be a relationship break-up where it is natural to feel depressed. They prescribe these drugs to people who are seriously depressed or it is a long standing problem. Anti-depressants may have to be taken for many months.

How Anti-Depressant Drugs Work

It is believed that these drugs work by increasing the activity of certain chemicals in the brain and thus producing a better mood.

Different Types of Anti-Depressants

There are different types of anti-depressants. Your GP will decide which anti-depressant to put you on. You will likely have a follow up meeting so your GP can see how you are feeling as a result of taking the tablets. They may change the dosage or the type of anti-depressant.

How Anti-Depressants Effect You

You can ask your GP how long the anti-depressant will take to work. Usually they take between 2 to 8 weeks. Even if you don't start to feel better it is very important that you do not stop taking the medication before seeing your GP. Your GP needs to manage your medication levels from start to finish. When you feel you no longer need the anti-depressants, please speak to your GP.

If you miss a dose, look at your anti-depressant medical leaflet for advice or call your GP. You can ask your GP in advance, what to do if you miss a dose.

Counselling

Counselling is advice and support given from a health professional. It is aimed at helping people with a particular problem. It may be to do with a physical illness, such as cancer or a mental illness such as depression. It is a good idea to seek some form of counselling as it can help enormously. You may find the first counsellor you try is not quite right for you but do not give up. Keep on trying until you find one suitable. Counselling is either on a one to one basis or in a group. Group therapy can be very beneficial as you get to meet people like yourself so you realise you are not alone and you can give each other advice and support plus you make new friends. However, if you have particular problems, which you know are causing your depression, then it is best if you have counselling on a one to one basis.

Your GP can sometimes send you to a counsellor for free depending on whether you meet certain criteria. However, there is usually a long waiting list for this service. You can also pay for a private counsellor. Price varies greatly from £25 an hour to £75 an hour. Make sure they are qualified.

Sorting Out Your Problems

In this chapter we are going to try to sort some of your problems out. We may not be able to sort all of them but at least by sorting a few of them some of the weight will be lifted off your mind. In some cases expert help may be needed i.e. when you are coping with a disturbing event. It may also be helpful to seek counselling for your problems, especially ones where you can see no way out. I would recommend counselling to anyone with depression but until you can afford it, or if you do not want to go, then this chapter will be very beneficial to you.

Do the following exercise when you have a good 1 ½ hrs to spare. Sit somewhere on your own in a quiet room where you will not be disturbed. It needs to be a place where you feel calm and relaxed. You will need a pen and some paper. Next I want you to write down all your problems, every last little one. Then follow the instructions very carefully that I have written below. We are going to code your problems in severity.

1. Put a star next to every problem you think is quite easily solved.

2. Now put circles next to ones which are difficult but you think they can be solved i.e. you will hopefully not be stuck with them for life. Write them down, no matter how painful, embarrassing and difficult they will be to solve.

3. Next underline the ones which are completely not solvable such as turning 20 or bringing a person or animal back to life.

We are going to start with the problems marked with a **star**. On a new piece of paper write one problem at the top of the page and carry on writing each problem at the top of the page until they are all done. Now follow these instructions.

1. Think very hard, take your time and write down any possible solutions. Leave an inch between each one. Even if you do not think you would have the guts to carry it through or it sounds crazy still write it down.

2. Read each one and imagine carrying each one through. Write under each solution things which could go wrong, the pros and cons, and a rating out of ten as to how good you think this solution is. Only do this if you think it is necessary to your particular problem.

3. Read through all the possible solutions to your problem. Judge each one on its effectiveness and put lines through all the solutions you think are not much good.

4. If you have a decision between a few solutions, it may help you to actually close your eyes and imagine the people and their personalities (if people are involved). If it is something you have got to say, say it out loud and in different tones of voice. Try to think when might be an appropriate time to speak to that person.

If your problem is not to do with anyone and is more of a personal problem maybe you could try a few solutions. Decide how much time you will give each one, bearing in mind you might not see a difference instantly. However, if one of your solutions is failing miserably then change it immediately. If your problem is an embarrassing medical problem it is very important you go to the doctors or chemist. They have seen it millions of times before. They are professionals. Remember, they do not know you. If they do know you and you are worried about it, go to a different doctor or chemist for this particular problem. If it is a sex problem which you may believe could be psychological then it may be helpful to talk to a counsellor. If you are too ashamed there are always telephone counsellors or online counsellors. Do not be afraid.

Next we are going to deal with the problems which are underlined. These are the problems that you cannot solve i.e. you cannot change them. To deal with these problems you need to find different ways of looking at them. For example, if you think you are not happy with your looks, write down all the things you like about yourself and all the things you think are okay. Next write down all the things that you do not have that you would hate to have. By doing this you will begin to realise how lucky you actually are. Also remember you cannot change it and worrying about it does not help, does it? No. It will just deepen your depression and make your recovery longer and we do not want that, do we? No. I know it is hard not to worry about it, especially when friends or family think it is funny to take the juice. Try to ignore them. A makeover is a good idea to boost your confidence or a new haircut.

If you are worried about turning a certain age, you can try to look at it from a more positive viewpoint. Think how long you have lived and the first five years you cannot remember much anyway. Also think how lucky you are, some people do not even make it to your age.

If your problem is that someone has died, it is important first of all that you grieve. This book does not go into detail about bereavement, so I suggest you read a special book on coping with bereavement if you think it may help. Professional help may also be of use to you. I know you probably think nothing will take your pain away and you are right it will not but it can give you ways to cope better. A nice way to remember someone or an animal is to make a scrap book of their life so you can remember the happy moments you both shared. Another positive thought is feeling privileged to have known them. You had the honour of sharing some of your life with them. You may want to plant a tree or flower in their memory. Remember they are always there in your memory.

If you have a serious illness counselling may help you cope.

There may be some problems which you had underlined which are now not as final as you first thought, however they do still seem difficult to solve. Mark these problems with an 'X'.

We are now going to move on to the problems marked with a circle. These are ones which are difficult, but possible, to solve i.e. they will not be here forever especially if we do something about them. I will warn you now these can be quite tricky to do.

1. Write each problem at the top of a new page as you did before.

2. Next to each problem on a scale of 1 to 10 (1 being least to 10 being max) rate how bad you consider it to be and how much it upsets you. Write just one number for each problem. We are going to deal with the easiest (lowest rated) first and work our way up.

3. Starting with your easiest problem (lowest rated) first, write down all the possible solutions for each one. Even if you think you could not do it, write it down.

4. Think really hard about each solution. Imagine carrying it out. How do you feel? How does it go? Write next to each how easily you would find it to carry out the solution. Use a scale of 1 to 10 (1 being very difficult 10 being fairly easy).

5. For each problem try the solutions which have the highest ratings.

Now to the problems marked with an 'X'. These are the hardest to solve, they are probably embarrassing problems or ones which you cannot face. I know it is hard. It may be leaving a dead end relationship and being scared to be on your own. You only have one life and if you are feeling partly depressed because of this problem then you have to break free. What is a few months of feeling hurt when you have freed your life up, well for life?

Your problem may be sex related and you are too embarrassed to seek help. Usually you know what to do about these problems. You need to go to the doctors, end that relationship, etc. If you feel you do not have the courage, then preparation is key. For example if you want to leave a relationship but you have kids and you feel can't leave, you may find reading relationship self-help books useful. You might decide to have counselling or seek professional advice. Emotionally prepare yourself. Work out what you will say to the people involved. Work out what you will do once you have told them. Work out what you will do to cope with your life in the immediate weeks or months afterwards. You might find absorbing yourself in socialising or a new hobby can help in this difficult time. Accept you might feel more emotional during this time.

Hopefully you now have some solutions or at least some ideas for how you are going to solve your problems that may be contributing to your depression. So start today and try some of these solutions.

You have done really well. Sorting out your problems is a big and difficult step and you are already half way there. Whatever you do, do not dismiss what you have just done. Do not put it to the back of a drawer and go back to your 'old ways'. If you still have problems you cannot solve, seek professional help.

Coping with Family, Friends and Events

Depression in its self is very hard to cope with. It is hard enough feeling the extreme hurt every day, the loneliness, the despair but what makes depression twice as hard to deal with is other people. Some of you may have friends or family who simply do not understand your illness. They might think that they understand your illness, but they don't. Sometimes what they say can make you feel really hurt and low.

Some people may grudgingly ask how you are and if you start to tell them they cut you short or you see their eyes glaze over. Some people may put you down by saying you'll always be like this and that is just who you are. Others may say hurtful things like 'so and so said they saw you the other day and you looked really grumpy'. Another line often heard is 'why don't you just cheer up'. If only it was that simple! These statements can really hurt you. I used to cry for hours on end when someone said something even slightly horrible to me. In the end you begin to dread speaking to these people let alone seeing them face to face as they can make you so angry and upset. You would ideally like to be able to brush off what they say but it is a lot easier said than done, When you do see these people face to face you may find yourself putting on a smiley face to say 'look I am happy, I can be happy too!'

These people are not bad people. It is not their fault they do not understand your illness. Try not to resent them too much and just dislike the fact that they simply do not understand. I know you may feel a lot of anger towards these people and this is understandable. You feel they have hurt you and made you feel bad. It can be difficult to understand what depression feels like when you have not experienced it yourself. Try to develop strategies to manage these situations. You might decide to not react to their comments and move the conversation on to something more positive. You might decide to try and explain your illness in a different way.

Another big problem you may find with depression is the upsetting feeling of letting others down. It especially happens when you have arranged to go out with friends or family and the thought of going out is too daunting. Whether it's the actual socialising or the energy needed the depressed person can find socialising very difficult. You may even feel you dread your own Birthday and all that your Birthday brings such as an increase in social engagements and lots of people directing their attention to you.

How to Cope with Friends, Family and Events

1. Seeing Friends and Family

I realise this is hard and although you may look forward to seeing your best mate and going for a game of football the reality of it can be very draining. One of the most important things I would say here is, to take off the pressure whenever and wherever you can. The less pressure you feel the more likely you are to look forward to it and the easier it will be to do. So how do we lessen the pressure?

You might find socialising with less people is easier for you. Alternatively, you might find a large group easier as it means less attention is on you. For example say there is 10 of you going out clubbing, if you do not turn up no one will be that annoyed as everyone else is there. However, saying this you may be the type of person who does not feel well in large groups and find it easier on a one to one basis. Work out what is easiest for you and act accordingly. Another good way to take the pressure off and to make sure you feel good is to arrange things at the latest possible minute. When you feel good, phone up your friends or family and ask to see them now or that night. Do it when you feel well.

Whatever you do, do make sure you try and see people even if you feel you cannot be bothered. It is important you keep a social life as much as possible. A social life, no matter how small, will give you support, encouragement and will make you laugh. It can be difficult to meet up with people when you feel low and it is usually the last thing you feel like doing but most of the time you will find if you make the effort and go out you do actually have quite a good time and it cheers you up. And this can't be bad can it? So do have a go. It is helpful to set yourself a target such as

I will go for an hour and then come home, but you will usually find yourself staying that little bit longer.

You may find that you no longer enjoy being around some of your friends as they make you feel bad about your depression. If you can't cope with them try seeing them a little less for a while, or arrange to meet up just for a quick coffee. See how you get on. You might find you lose some friends when you are suffering with depression. This happened to me. I lost one of my best friends. However, I met up with her by chance years later and we have been best friends again ever since. It wasn't her fault she didn't understand my illness, we were only teenagers at the time.

You may be lucky enough to have people in your life who want to learn and understand your illness. For these people do explain how you feel, what makes you feel good and bad and how they can help. I found these people appreciated being thanked. Sometimes I just thanked them, other times I got them a small card. These people are great to have by side during your recovery.

2. Special Events

By special events I am talking about weddings, birthdays, parties, Christmas, New Year etc. These can be tricky. It is a special event so everybody is expecting you to be there. It is a special event so you are expected to be happy. In these circumstances you may feel under pressure and wish you did not have to go. But you must at least try if not for your own sake, then for others. Even if you go just for a couple of hours it shows that you have tried.

If you really feel that you cannot go still try to celebrate the event. If for instance it was a friend's Birthday and you did not feel up to going out for the meal, make your apologies and then send her a Birthday card to arrive on the day. It shows you care and it is your illness that is stopping you. If it is a really special event such as a wedding then try really hard to go. Accept you will probably feel awful but ignore it to the best of your ability. At least if you try to go, people will see that you are at least trying.

In these circumstances if you think you may not be able to attend, tell them in advance. Explain due to your illness you may not be able to make it but you will try your hardest.

3. Partners

I hope for your sake your partner understands your illness. If they do it will make your recovery so much easier. If they do not it can be terrible and impact negatively on your relationship. It can be so emotionally draining and you will probably find yourself having endless arguments. This must be sorted out.

For a start ask them to read this:

You partner has an illness. It is just like any other illness, it takes time to get better and they need your support. They need you to look after them just as much as if it was a physical illness. Depression occurs when there is a chemical imbalance in the brain. 1 in 4 people will get it at least once in their lives. Yes! Even you! So maybe you could take an hour or so out of your schedule and read some of this book, particularly the chapter 'What Depression Feels Like' or even talk to your partner for half an hour and actually listen to what they are telling you. It is invaluable. Try not to interrupt with your views. I know it is hard but it is the worst thing you can do. Please give your partner this time. It will mean a lot to them and will make it easier for both of you. Secondly I know it is hard to cope with and you may feel at the end of your tether, but be there for them and the recovery will be a lot quicker and less painless. Ask your partner what they want you to do. Thank you for taking the time to read this.

Eating Well and Exercise

We constantly hear day in and day out that we are supposed to eat healthily and do plenty of exercise to prevent various diseases. But we are young so what do we care? Well you may not care but, as I am sure some of you would agree, we should care.

Many people are conscious of their weight. Advertisements, magazines and television show us we should be stick thin or muscular. This can make us get anxious about our size which in turn can lead us to comfort eat to make ourselves feel better. This then makes us gain weight and then we have to go on countless diets which we ultimately give up on. We can then end up comforting eating. It is a viscous cycle. The best way is to eat healthily with the odd treat and do plenty of exercise

Eating well and exercising actually makes you feel good and if you feel good then your depression will lift. It's okay to have treats now and again. There is lots of information on healthy eating on the internet. The NHS website has healthy eating guidelines.

Exercise is extremely important when recovering from depression. It releases feel good chemicals into the brain. This will help to create a sense of well being and provide you with a sense of achievement. It also provides purpose and it can be very good fun. The thing I must stress here is that you do an exercise you enjoy. If you don't enjoy the exercise you may feel more inclined to give up. So the first task is to find an exercise you will enjoy.

First decide if you want to exercise alone. There are advantages and disadvantages for exercising in a group or individually.

Exercising in a Group

More fun, others encourage you, shared costs, social activity (might meet new friends), safe. The disadvantages are that others may let you down, you do not concentrate as much, there are distractions, you have to exercise at set times, you have to go to the designated place. You have to decide which is best for you. You may want to try out a few activities before you find the one or two you want to stick at.

Some ideas for group sports include tennis, basketball, netball, squash, aerobics, running, dancing, volleyball, mountain biking (off road), badminton.

Sole Activities for Exercise

Individual sports you could do include swimming, home aerobics, running, dancing, bike riding, walking, horse riding, gym, weight training.

There are many more. Why not pop into your local sports centre and pick up a leaflet.

As you are depressed you may think exercise is a waste of time. 'What's the point? I'm fit enough already. I don't have the time. I've got better things to do! I don't feel like it!' These are all reasons for not doing exercise. I want you to try exercising for two weeks and then see if you feel any better. I think you will find that you do.

How much should you exercise?

½ hour a day
½ hour every other day
1 hour every other day

It is up to you! The NHS provides advice on the amount of exercise you should do. Take a look at their website. Even if you start doing just a little exercise, it is better than doing nothing.

Remember you can bring exercise into everyday life. You could cycle to your friends instead of taking the bus, walk places instead of taking the car and dance in a club or around your bedroom.

When should you exercise?

Whenever is best for you. Make sure you do not exercise on a full stomach or an empty one. It is best to eat an hour beforehand or just eat something light and wait 20 minutes for it to go down.

Exercise will help you on your way to recovery and what way could your time be better spent? Exercise is a great healer and will take away some of the pain. Look at it as a medicine. Do it for you. Now. Start today. Go on. You can do it.

Exercise is also a great way to get frustration and anger out of our system. Feel yourself sweating tension and stress out of your body.

Once again there is lots of information on fitness and different activities you can do on the NHS website.

Healing Through Self-Nurturance

So you take care of others. You look after them when they are ill without even thinking about it. You tell them to rest, take it easy and eat well. But since when have you looked after yourself? No, I mean really when? Chances are you forget about yourself, as it does not seem important. Looking after yourself may seem a waste of time but I assure you it is not. In fact it is a very nice and valuable way to spend your time right now.

Self-nurturance i.e. looking after yourself, indulging yourself and having treats has a lot to answer for. Do not rely on others to make you feel special, make yourself feel special. Treat yourself. It is also a great way of healing your mind and body, which is one of the things you need right now. By healing your body you will gain strength, confidence and the will to go forwards. You will experience happiness and a lot of comfort. What more could you ask for? Self-nurturance is a vital tool in recovering from depression and indeed anxiety. It will revive you and remind you there are some nice things in this world and you can feel good.

By now I should have convinced you! So what can you do to self-nurture yourself? It can be a small or large thing. It may be as small as making a cup tea and enjoying a bar of chocolate while watching your favourite television programme. It could be having a deep warm bath with your nicest bubble bath, reading a magazine or listening to the radio. One of my favourite ways to self-nurture was to hire out a video and indulge in just cooked cakes. Some find retail therapy good. Buy a computer game or some flowers (unless you have financial worries). It is really anything you enjoy but there is one important rule - IT MUST BE SOLO. I know a lot of you spend a lot of time on your own and I also know how much this can hurt, so you are probably thinking, 'How can I enjoy something on my own? I will hurt so what is the point?' The point is a) prove you can enjoy yourself on your own b) to make you actually like being on your own sometimes and c) if you share the experience it is not as healing. By all means you can nurture yourself with others and it will help you too but it is not as effective as if you were on your own.

The way you use self-nurturance is completely up to you. You may like to use it as a reward. For example, you look back on your day and realise how well you have done so you treat yourself. You might use self-nurturance as an encourager for example, plan that after a meal with the relatives you will treat yourself to a movie. Another way is to use it in setback as a healer and comforter. Look at it as free medication that is going to make you feel better and help you on your road to recovery. It should definitely be in your plan of recovery or at the very least in your tool box! Use it as and when you feel like it. You do not need a reason!

Another way of looking after your self is not to mentally beat yourself up as so many of us do. Often you may find yourself thinking what a horrible person you are and how you can't do anything right. Try to ignore these feelings. Say to yourself I feel like this because of my illness and when I get better these feelings will lessen. Forget them for now, they are not important. If you can, be kind to yourself and recovery will be so much quicker and easier. What does feeling guilty and upset achieve? Nothing. All it does is prolong your recovery. So what is the best thing to do? Think about it. Thought about it? You probably realised it is pointless to make yourself feel bad. Of course you may feel a bit guilty and low at times, and that is to be expected, but don't make it even harder on yourself. Just get on with whatever it is you are doing.

The same applies to Setback. What does fretting about it actually achieve? Just take some time out, indulge yourself in whatever you fancy and rest. You can read this book again, no matter how many times you have before. Then you can start fresh again. Remember, any achievements no matter how small will always 'count'. You NEVER go back to the beginning. You only ever drop a bit behind – remember the setback diagram? So remember be kind to yourself.

Music & Writing

Music

Listening to music can be an excellent way to help you in your recovery. You can use it in many different ways, as an uplifter, comforter, release of tension or a reminder. When exercising put on a jumpy, dance music, it has to be something you really enjoy. It will make you feel good and you will enjoy the exercise so much more. Your spirits will be higher. You can use an uplifting song to lift your mood whenever you want.

You might find a song that relates to how you feel and this can act as a great comforter. Listen to it when you want to be reminded that you are not alone and others out there are feeling exactly the same as you.

Find a song that is nice and relaxing. An album is best as you can leave it to play on and on. Play it softly or play it loud and completely let your mind be absorbed in the music. You could listen to the album whilst in a candle lit bath or while you are reading a book.

Try to find an encouraging song. Try to find one with lines that refer to things getting brighter in the future. Anything that makes you feel better about the future is great.

Writing

There are three ways of using writing as a tool towards recovery.

Please note: Hide away any writings in an extremely safe place or throw them away. (Do not throw no. 3 away.)

1. Write out exactly how you feel, what makes you feel bad, who makes you feel bad, how you wish it was different and then write ways in which you could help the matter or deal with it better.

2. Use it to voice opinions or anger on somebody and release all the tension through your writing. You could even write it in the form of a

letter telling them exactly what you think of them. Do not, whatever you do, send it.

3. Some of you may feel a lot of confusion about what life is all about. You might spend time wondering what people want in a friend or a girlfriend/boyfriend. So make a book and write it down so you do not have to keep going over it in your head as you have written it all down. It really clears your head out.

Good Things That Come Out of Depression

In the midst of Depression you wouldn't believe that anything good could actually come out of it, But as you start to get better you realise, 'Hey. It was horrible but I am a better, stronger person than I was before.' Not only that but all this as well:

1. You know yourself better.
2. You give up putting on an act all of the time to please others.
3. More realistic views on life.
4. More realistic views on the world.
5. You are more understanding and sympathetic towards others. If they have a problem you will find 9 times out of 10 they will come to you, which really bonds your friendship
6. You are more at ease.
7. Feel content.
8. More ambitious but at the same time realistic.
9. You learn to exercise and eat well.
10. Know how to control stress.
11. Know how to release tension.
12. Enjoy the simpler, freer things in life.
13. Can reason with yourself and others.
14. Can solve most problems and know how to deal with things.
15. Know that running away from your problems actually makes them worse. The only way to get rid of them is to face up to them.
16. Gain new interests and hobbies.
17. Gain new friends from help groups or exercise groups.
18. You sort out your views and principles.
19. Become a good listener.
20. You become a good helper.
21. You eventually have more confidence in yourself.
22. Last but definitely the most important, you learn how to make yourself happier than ever before.

Keeping Out of Depression

1. Remember and practice what you have learned.
2. Let yourself back into normal life slowly.
3. Be content with what you have got, many people are not as lucky as you.
4. Remember others lives are not always what they seem. You do not know what goes on behind closed doors. Very few people in this life have everything they want.
5. Know you do not have to be happy all the time. Everyone has down days. Be yourself.
6. If you have a problem face it, sort it out. Never run away.
7. If you are not happy with something, have the courage to change it.
8. If you are feeling tense, take time out to relax.
9. Play your uplifting tunes every now and then as a bit of therapy.
10. Boost self-esteem occasionally by having a new look, hairstyle, top etc.
11. Have something to do and something to look forward to.
12. Do not be depressed just to get attention, gain attention for your positive emotions.
13. Take life less seriously. Remember to laugh.
14. Help others.
15. Have time to yourself to relax once a week.
16. Take care of yourself in every sense of the word. (Self-Nurturance.)
17. If you feel yourself starting to slip back, re-read this book.
18. Realise how great you are!

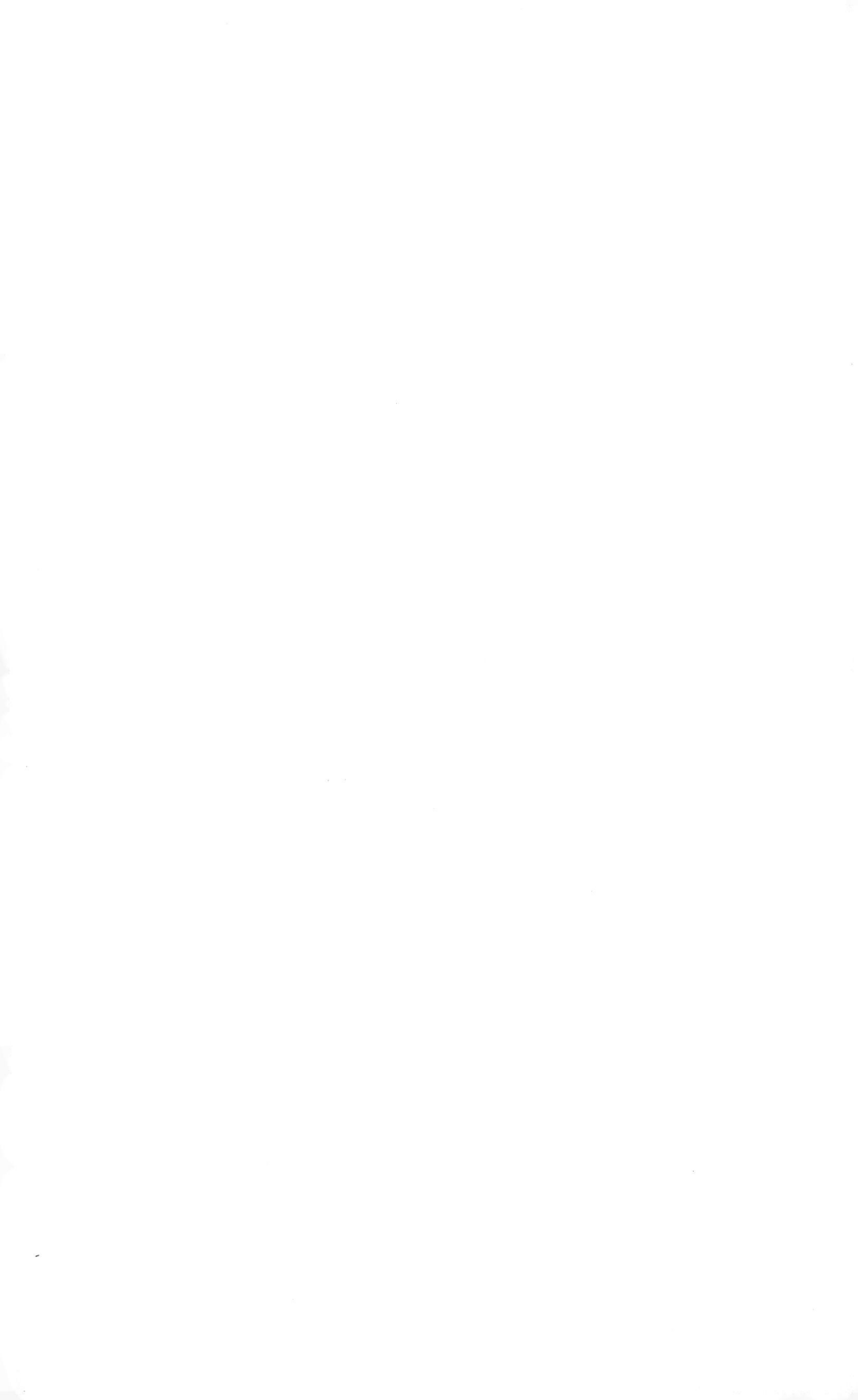

Printed in Great Britain
by Amazon.co.uk, Ltd.,
Marston Gate.